JENNY BEADLE

12 Weeks of High-Intensity Strength Training

Intense Sessions to Build Muscle, Increase Metabolism, and Sculpt Your Body from Head to Toe

First edition

This book was professionally typeset on Reedsy.
Find out more at reedsy.com

Contents

Introduction

Welcome to Your Transformation

Congratulations on taking the first step toward building a stronger, healthier, and more confident you! Whether you're a seasoned fitness enthusiast or someone just starting your journey, this program is designed to help you achieve lasting results. Strength training isn't just about lifting weights; it's about unlocking your potential, enhancing your everyday life, and reshaping your relationship with your body and mind.

This book is your guide to a 12-week high-intensity strength training program that's challenging, effective, and empowering. By following the plan laid out here, you'll build muscle, increase your metabolism, and sculpt your body from head to toe.

Why a 12-Week Program?

In fitness, consistency is key. Results don't happen overnight, but they do happen when you commit to a structured, well-designed plan. Twelve weeks is the perfect time frame to build strength, develop new habits, and see visible changes in your body. This isn't a quick-fix program or a crash diet—it's a sustainable approach to fitness that lays the foundation for long-term health and strength.

Overview of the Program Structure

This 12-week program includes a total of 12 unique workouts, one for each week. You'll complete the workout of the week, (WOW), three times during that week, focusing on mastering the movements and progressively increasing your strength, speed, and/or duration. This repetition allows you to track your progress and build confidence with each exercise.

Each workout is designed to target your entire body, with a mix of compound movements (like squats and deadlifts) and isolation exercises (like bicep curls and tricep extensions), and some high intensity movements to keep your heart rate elevated. These exercises are carefully balanced to ensure you're working all major muscle groups while giving your body the recovery it needs to grow stronger.

In addition to physical progress, you'll also track metrics such as weight lifted, workout duration, and the number of repetitions or rounds completed. Tracking these details is a critical part of your success—it allows you to see how far you've come and motivates you to keep pushing forward.

This program is adaptable for all fitness levels. If you're a beginner, you'll find detailed instructions and modifications to help you get started safely. If you're more advanced, you'll appreciate the focus on progression and the opportunity to push your limits.

So, are you ready to commit to a program that will transform your body and mind? Let's get started! Your strongest self is just 12 weeks away.

1

Chapter 1: The Benefits of Strength Training

Introduction to Strength Training Benefits

Strength training is one of the most transformative activities you can include in your fitness journey. It isn't just about lifting weights or achieving a sculpted physique; it's about creating a stronger, healthier, and more capable version of yourself. Whether you're a seasoned athlete, a busy parent, or someone completely new to exercise, strength training can benefit everyone. From improving everyday functionality to enhancing your mental well-being, the rewards of resistance training extend far beyond the gym.

What is Strength Training?

At its core, strength training involves using resistance to improve the strength, endurance, and size of muscles. This resistance can come from free weights, machines, resistance bands, or even your own body weight. Exercises like squats, push-ups, deadlifts, and rows challenge your muscles to work harder than usual, which leads to growth and adaptation. Unlike some forms of exercise that focus solely on calorie burn or flexibility, strength training builds the foundation for overall fitness, supporting cardiovascular health, mobility, and durability.

Building Muscle and Strength

The Role of Muscle in Everyday Function and Performance
Your muscles are essential for nearly every movement you make. From climbing stairs to lifting grocery bags, they play a vital role in maintaining your independence and quality of life. Stronger muscles mean greater ease and efficiency in everyday tasks. Beyond that, muscle strength enhances athletic performance, allowing you to run faster, jump higher, or swing harder, depending on your sport or hobby.

How Increased Strength Improves Quality of Life
Imagine not having to struggle with heavy luggage, feeling confident playing with your children or grandchildren, or reducing back pain caused by weak muscles. Strength training translates to real-world improvements that make life more enjoyable and less physically taxing. It's not just about physical power; it's about empowering yourself to tackle daily challenges with confidence.

Increasing Metabolism and Burning Fat

The Relationship Between Muscle Mass and Resting Metabolic Rate (RMR)

Muscle isn't just active tissue when you're working out—it's a calorie-burning powerhouse even at rest. For every pound of muscle you gain, your body burns more calories throughout the day, boosting your resting metabolic rate (RMR). This means that even while you're sitting or sleeping, your body is working harder to maintain itself.

Why Strength Training is More Effective Than Cardio Alone for Long-Term Fat Loss

While cardiovascular exercise burns calories during a workout, strength training offers a twofold benefit: it burns calories during exercise and helps you build muscle that continues to burn calories long afterward. Additionally, the process of muscle repair after strength training, known as excess post-exercise oxygen consumption (EPOC), keeps your metabolism elevated for hours. Combined, these factors make strength training a cornerstone of sustainable fat loss.

Enhancing Bone Density and Joint Health

How Resistance Training Combats Osteoporosis

Bone health becomes increasingly important as we age, particularly for women at risk of osteoporosis. Resistance training stimulates bone remodeling, increasing bone density and reducing the risk of fractures. The stress applied to bones during weight-bearing exercises triggers their natural rebuilding process, making them stronger over time.

The Impact of Muscle Strength on Joint Stability and Injury Prevention

Strong muscles provide better support for your joints, reducing the likelihood of injuries. For example, strengthening the quadriceps and hamstrings protects your knees, while building core strength supports your spine. This improved stability allows for safer movement patterns in everyday activities and reduces wear and tear on joints, particularly for those with arthritis or joint pain.

Mental and Emotional Benefits

Stress Reduction Through Endorphin Release

Exercise, including strength training, is a natural stress reliever. Physical activity triggers the release of endorphins—your body's feel-good chemicals—that elevate your mood and reduce feelings of anxiety or depression. Strength training can also serve as a form of mindfulness, focusing your attention on the present moment as you concentrate on your form, breathing, and movement.

Improved Self-Confidence and Body Image

There's something empowering about lifting weights and realizing your strength is growing. Strength training can improve your self-esteem and body image, not necessarily because of physical changes but because of the sense of accomplishment and resilience it fosters. Feeling capable and strong translates into other areas of life, boosting confidence in ways that extend beyond the gym.

Long-Term Health Benefits

Reducing Risks of Chronic Illnesses
Regular strength training can lower your risk of chronic conditions like type 2 diabetes, heart disease, and hypertension. Increased muscle mass improves insulin sensitivity, helping regulate blood sugar levels, while the act of resistance training strengthens the cardiovascular system.

Improving Mobility and Independence as You Age
As we grow older, maintaining muscle mass becomes crucial for staying active and independent. Strength training helps combat sarcopenia—the age-related loss of muscle mass—and keeps you mobile. This means you can continue doing the things you love, from gardening to traveling, without physical limitations.

Conclusion: Why Start Today?

Strength training isn't just exercise; it's an investment in your future self. By building muscle, boosting metabolism, and protecting your joints, you're setting the stage for a healthier, more resilient body. The mental clarity and emotional strength you'll gain are just as rewarding.

This 12-week program is designed to make strength training accessible, effective, and enjoyable. Whether you're starting from scratch or looking to enhance your routine, there's no better time to begin. Your stronger, healthier future is just a few reps away.

2

Chapter 2: The Science Behind Strength Training

Strength training may seem straightforward—lift weights, get stronger—but the process driving those results is complex and fascinating. To make the most of your workouts, it's essential to understand the science behind how muscles grow, how to structure your training sessions, and the principles that lead to continuous progress.

How Muscles Grow: Hypertrophy Explained

At the heart of strength training is **hypertrophy**, the process by which muscles increase in size. When you lift weights, you create small tears in your muscle fibers. This might sound counterproductive, but these micro-tears are essential for muscle growth. During recovery, your body repairs these tears by fusing fibers together and adding new muscle tissue. Over time, this process makes your muscles stronger and larger.

Hypertrophy is influenced by three primary factors:

1. **Mechanical Tension:** This is the tension your muscles

experience when lifting weights. Exercises like squats, bench presses, and deadlifts generate significant tension, especially when performed with proper form and heavy loads.

2. **Muscle Damage:** Those small tears mentioned earlier are a form of controlled damage. This damage signals your body to initiate repair and growth processes. While some soreness after a workout is normal, excessive pain can indicate overtraining or improper form.

3. **Metabolic Stress:** The burning sensation you feel during high-rep sets is an example of metabolic stress. This occurs when your muscles work under conditions of limited oxygen, creating a buildup of byproducts like lactic acid. This stress is another signal to your body that it's time to adapt and grow stronger.

To optimize hypertrophy, your workouts need to balance these factors. Too much damage or insufficient tension can stall progress. By following a structured plan like this 12-week program, you'll create the perfect environment for muscle growth.

Understanding the Lingo

The workouts in this program are based on a variety of training methods designed to increase your strength, speed, and endurance. Each one plays a specific role in determining your workout's intensity and focus.

1. **Repetitions (Reps):** A rep is one complete movement of an exercise. For example, lowering and lifting a barbell during a bench press counts as one rep.

2. **Rounds:** This refers to the entire circuit that is written. For example, if the workout is 10 exercises, completed in succession as a circuit, and you do the circuit three times, you have completed 3 rounds.

3. **EMOM:** Every Minute on the Minute - This refers to the cadence in which you will complete a particular series of exercises. If it says "Do 20 reps of sit-ups EMOM", it means do 20 sit-ups and then rest for the remainder of that minute. When the next minute starts, do it again.

4. **AMRAP:** As Many Rounds As Possible - This means you should complete the circuit as many times as possible in the allotted time. This program combines strength training with high intensity intervals for maximum fat loss, so time is an important factor.

- NOTE - Some workouts in this series will use AMRAP for "As Many Reps As Possible", meaning do as many repetitions as possible in the allotted time. Be sure to pay attention to this!

1. **Rest Periods:** The time you take between exercises or rounds can influence your workout's effectiveness. Each workout indicates the appropriate rest period for you.

The Role of Progressive Overload

If you want to see continuous progress, one principle stands above all others: **progressive overload**. This concept refers to gradually increasing the demands placed on your muscles over time. Without progressive overload, your body has no reason to adapt, and your progress will plateau.

Progressive overload can be achieved in several ways:

1. **Increasing Weight:** The most common method is to lift heavier weights. For example, if you start bench pressing 100 pounds, increasing to 105 pounds over a few weeks challenges your muscles to adapt.
2. **Adding Reps or Sets:** If increasing weight isn't feasible, adding more reps or sets to your workouts also increases the workload. For instance, performing 12 reps instead of 10 or doing an additional set adds volume to your training.
3. **Improving Technique:** Focusing on better form, controlled movements, and a full range of motion can make an exercise more challenging without adding weight.
4. **Reducing Rest Periods:** Shortening rest intervals forces your muscles to work harder within a given time frame, increasing the intensity of your workout.
5. **Increasing Time Under Tension:** Slowing down the eccentric (lowering) phase of a lift or holding a contraction for longer increases the strain on your muscles, promoting growth.

Progressive overload doesn't mean you have to make drastic changes every session. Small, consistent increases in weight or workload are enough to keep your muscles adapting. Tracking your progress is key; writing down the weights, reps, and sets you complete in each workout helps ensure you're continuously challenging yourself.

Putting It All Together

Now that you understand how muscles grow, and the importance of progressive overload, you're equipped with the knowledge to maximize your results. This program is designed to incorporate these principles seamlessly, guiding you through a progression that challenges your muscles while giving them the time they need to recover and grow.

Let's move forward with confidence, knowing that every lift, every set, and every drop of effort is a step closer to your goals. The science behind strength training isn't just theory—it's the foundation for the transformation you're about to experience.

3

Chapter 3: Setting Your Goals and Tracking Progress

Goal setting and progress tracking are two of the most critical aspects of a successful strength training journey. Without a clear vision of where you want to go and a system to measure your progress, it's easy to lose motivation or plateau. In this chapter, we'll walk through how to set realistic goals, measure your starting point, and track your workouts and milestones. By the end, you'll have a roadmap to guide your 16-week transformation and beyond.

Establishing Realistic Goals

Before you dive into your first workout, it's essential to define what you want to achieve. Are you looking to build muscle, increase strength, improve endurance, lose fat, or a combination of these? Your goals will shape how you approach the program and the metrics you focus on tracking.

1. **Specific Goals:** Avoid vague objectives like "I want to get

fit." Instead, set precise targets such as "I want to bench press 150 pounds," "I want to lose 10 pounds of fat," or "I want to perform 20 consecutive push-ups." Specific goals give you clarity and direction.

2. **Measurable Goals:** Ensure your goals are quantifiable so you can track progress. Use numbers, time frames, or other metrics to define success. For example, "I want to lose 20 pounds in 12 weeks" is measurable.

3. **Achievable Goals:** While ambition is great, setting unattainable goals can lead to frustration. Consider your starting point, lifestyle, and available time. A beginner might aim to improve their overall strength, while an experienced lifter might focus on adding 5-10% to their lifts.

4. **Relevant Goals:** Align your goals with your personal motivations. If improving functional strength for everyday activities matters most to you, find a way to measure that. If you're more interested in weight loss or aesthetics of your body, find a way to measure that!

5. **Time-Bound Goals:** Goals without deadlines lack urgency. The 12-week program provides a built-in timeline, but you can break it down further. For example, you could set smaller goals to achieve at the end of each 4-week period.

Take some time to write down your goals. Be honest with yourself about what you want to achieve and why. Your goals should inspire and motivate you, serving as a reminder of why you started this journey.

Measuring Your Starting Point

Before embarking on any fitness program, it's crucial to establish a baseline. Knowing where you're starting from helps you track improvements and celebrate progress along the way.

1. **Body Measurements:** Use a tape measure to record key metrics such as:

- Chest
- Waist
- Hips
- Thighs
- Arms

Take measurements at the same time of day (e.g., in the morning) to ensure consistency.

1. **Body Weight and Composition:** Step on a scale to record your weight, but don't rely solely on this number. If possible, use body fat calipers, a smart scale, or a DEXA scan to determine your body fat percentage. Tracking changes in muscle mass versus fat mass provides a more accurate picture of your progress.
2. **Strength and Endurance Tests:** Test your current fitness levels with simple exercises:

- Maximum push-ups you can do in one set.
- Hold long you can hold a plank
- Number of reps at a moderate weight for an endurance benchmark.

1. **Flexibility and Mobility Assessments:** Assessing your

range of motion can help identify areas to work on. Can you touch your toes? How deep is your squat? Improved mobility can enhance performance and reduce injury risk.

Record all these measurements in a dedicated journal or digital app. These baseline numbers will serve as a reference point, highlighting your progress as you move through the program.

Tracking Workouts and Milestones

Once your goals are set and your starting point is measured, the next step is to track your workouts consistently. Tracking not only keeps you accountable but also allows you to make adjustments when necessary.

1. **Create a Workout Log:** Your workout log can be as simple or detailed as you like. At a minimum, record:

- The workout you performed and the date you completed it
- The weights you used for the various exercises
- The number of rounds and/or repetitions
- Rest periods that you took

1. **Monitor Progress Over Time:** Use progress photos to visualize your journey. Take progress photos every four weeks. Wear the same clothing and use consistent lighting and angles for accurate comparisons.
2. **Reflect on Non-Physical Achievements:** Strength training is as much about mental and emotional growth as it is about physical changes. Take note of improvements like increased confidence, reduced stress, or better focus.
3. **Adjust When Necessary:** If progress stalls, don't panic.

Plateaus are a natural part of any fitness journey. Review your workout logs to identify areas for improvement. Are you challenging yourself with progressive overload? Are your rest periods too short or too long? Adjust your training variables as needed.

Putting It All Together

By establishing realistic goals, measuring your starting point, and tracking your workouts, you're setting yourself up for success in this 12-week program. This process ensures that every step you take is intentional and measurable, bringing you closer to your goals.

As you move through the program, revisit your goals and measurements regularly. Celebrate your progress, no matter how small, and stay focused on the journey ahead. With dedication, consistency, and the right tools, your transformation is not just possible—it's inevitable. Let's get started!

4

Chapter 4: Essential Safety Guidelines

Strength training is an incredibly rewarding activity, but it requires the right tools and practices to ensure success and safety. Whether you're training at a fully equipped gym or creating a space at home, prioritizing proper form, and including essential warm-ups and mobility work are key to achieving your goals while avoiding injuries.

Proper Form and Injury Prevention

Good form is the foundation of effective strength training. Performing exercises correctly maximizes results and minimizes the risk of injury.

1. **Master the Basics First:** Before increasing weight, duration, or speed, focus on nailing the mechanics of each movement.
2. **Maintain Neutral Alignment:**

- Keep your spine neutral during lifts; avoid rounding or over-arching your back.

- Engage your core to stabilize your body.
- Ensure your knees track over your toes during lower body movements.

1. **Lift Within Your Limits:** Avoid ego lifting—choosing weights that are too heavy for your current strength level. This often leads to compromised form. Progress gradually as your strength increases.
2. **Listen to Your Body:** Pain and fatigue are signals that something may be off. If you feel discomfort during an exercise, stop immediately and assess your form or adjust the weight.

Injury prevention is a combination of proper technique, manageable intensity, and consistent recovery. A focus on these areas will keep you training effectively for the long term.

Warm-Ups, Cool-Downs, and Mobility Work

Strength training isn't just about the main workout. Preparing your body with a proper warm-up and aiding recovery with cool-downs and mobility work are critical to optimizing performance and reducing the risk of injury.

1. **Warm-Ups:** Warming up increases blood flow, raises body temperature, and prepares your muscles for the workout ahead.

- **Dynamic Stretching:** Movements like leg swings, arm circles, or spinal twists improve joint mobility.
- **Light Cardio:** 5–10 minutes of jogging, cycling, or jumping jacks gets your heart rate up.

- **Movement-Specific Drills:** Perform lighter versions of the exercises in your workout. For example, do bodyweight squats before weighted squats.

1. **Cool-Downs:**After your workout, cool-downs help reduce muscle soreness and aid recovery.

- **Static Stretching:** Hold stretches for major muscle groups (hamstrings, quads, chest) for 20–30 seconds.
- **Breathing Exercises:** Deep, slow breaths lower your heart rate and promote relaxation.

1. **Mobility Work:**Improved mobility enhances your range of motion, leading to better performance and reduced injury risk.

- **Foam Rolling:** Use a foam roller to release tight muscles and improve blood flow.
- **Joint Mobility Exercises:** Incorporate movements like hip circles or wrist stretches to keep joints healthy.
- **Yoga or Pilates:** These practices can supplement your strength training by enhancing flexibility and stability.

Consistency with warm-ups, cool-downs, and mobility work is just as important as consistency with your main workout routine.

Putting It All Together

Prioritizing proper form, and incorporating warm-ups and mobility work are all essential to a successful and safe strength training journey. Whether you're working out in a gym or at home, taking these precautions will help you achieve your goals while minimizing setbacks.

By creating a strong foundation, you'll not only build a stronger body but also set yourself up for long-term success. Remember: every effective workout begins with preparation and ends with care. Now that you have these tools, you're ready to tackle the program with confidence and focus.

5

Chapter 5: 12 Weeks of Workouts

The next 12 pages include your weekly workouts. Each workout should be completed 3 times during that week, with at least one day in between.

For example, each weeks' workout could be performed on Mon/Weds/Fri or Tues/Thurs/Sat.

You can include additional workouts on the other days if you like.

Be sure to track each workout in your chosen tracker. This could be a physical workout journal, an app, or a file on your tablet or computer. Just be sure to track your data. Refer back to chapter three if you don't recall what should be tracked.

LET'S GOOOO!!!

6

Week One: The Nasty Thirty

AMRAP (rounds) in 30 minutes: Complete as many rounds as possible of the following circuit in 30 minutes:

30 Box Jumps or DB Step Ups
  30 Burpees
  30 Kettlebell Swings
  30 Walking Lunges
  30 Pulsating Squats
  30 Push Presses
  30 Dumbbell Deadlifts
  30 Medicine Ball Slams
  30 1 leg Up Push-Ups
  30 Plank to Push-Ups

7

Week Two: Abzilla

EMOM, *5 Rounds:* Complete the following exercises every minute on the minute. If you finish before the minute is over, rest until the next one begins. Complete 5 rounds.

Min 1: 20 Bicycle Crunches (1 on each side = 1 rep)
   Min 2: 20 V-Ups
   Min 3: 40 Flutter Kicks (1 on each side = 1 rep)
   Min 4: 10 Burpees
   Min 5: 20 Knee-to-Chest Kickouts
   Min 6: Rest

8

Week Three: The Bambi

10 Rounds for Time: Complete the following circuit 10 times as quickly as possible. Each round should be completed in 3 minutes or less. Rest 1 minute between rounds.

21 Heavy Dumbbell Squats
  15 Jump Squats
  9 Heavy Dumbbell Deadlifts
  5 Overhead Medicine Ball Squats

9

Week Four: 21 Gunz Street

A MRAP *(reps) in 60 on/30 off, 2 rounds:* Complete 2 rounds of the following. Perform each exercise for 1 minute, and rest for 30 seconds between exercises.

Cross Body Curls
  Hammer Curls
  Tricep Extensions
  Alternating Dumbbell Curls
  Skull Crushers
  5 Count Bicep Curl Up
  5 Count Bicep Curl Down
  Tricep dips
  Diamond Push-Ups
  Curl & Press
  Tricep Kickbacks
  Pulsating Tricep Dip
  Pulsating Diamond Push-Ups
  Plank to Push-Ups

10

Week Five: One More Rep

AMRAP *(reps) in 45 on/15 off, 3 rounds:* Complete each exercise as follows: As many reps as possible in 45 seconds on, then 15 seconds to transition to the next exercise. Complete all 10 exercises and take 1 minute of rest between rounds. Complete three rounds.

Dumbbell Squats
    Bench Press (On Floor in Bridge position)
    Bent Over Rows
    Alternating Curtsy Lunges
    Shoulder Press
    Deadlifts
    Hammer Curls
    Tricep Overhead Extension
    Hip Bridges
    C Seated Lateral Raises

11

Week Six: Jump Around

Three Rounds for Time: Complete the following circuit 3 times. Rest as needed. Complete 20 Jumping Jacks between each exercise.

15 Thrusters
15 Sumo Deadlifts
15 Push Press
15 (each side) Alternating dumbbell snatches
15 DB Step-Ups
15 (each side) Renegade Rows
15 Goblet Squats
15 Burpees

12

Week Seven: Jack & Jill

A *MRAP (rounds), 20 minutes:* Complete as many rounds as possible in 20 minutes of the following circuit.

15 (each side) Single Arm Thrusters
15 DB Snatches
15 (each side) Bulgarian Split Squats
15 (each side) Renegade Rows
20 Goblet Squats

13

Week Eight: Eagle Eye

4 Rounds for Time: Complete 4 rounds as fast as possible of the following circuit:

20 (each side) Single-Arm DB Bent Over Row to Press
   20 (each side) One Arm Swings
   20 (each side) Single Leg Deadlifts
   20 (each side) Single Arm Snatch
   20 (each side) Front Lunge to Curls

14

Week Nine: Sweat Fest

EMOM, 30 Rounds, Active Rest Between Rounds: Complete the following exercises every minute on the minute. If you complete the reps before the minute is up, do push-ups for the remainder of that minute for odd minutes and mountain climbers for the remainder of the minute for even minutes.

2 (each side) Turkish Get Ups
   10 (each side) Woodchoppers
   25 Pull Overs
   25 Cleans
   25 Skull Crushers (in hollow hold position)
   25 Arnold Press
   25 DB Hip Bridges
   25 Tricep Kickbacks
   25 Alternating Reverse Lunges
   25 Rear Delt Flies

15

Week Ten: Walk This Weigh

MRAP (rounds) in 30 minutes: Complete as many rounds as possible in 25 minutes of the following circuit:

15 Overhead Squats
15 Power Burpee (Pushup, Curl, Press with Dumbbells)
15 Curl, to Press, to Triceps Extension
20 Bent Over Rows (reverse grip)
20 Suitcase Squats to Curls
2 Laps of Farmer's Carries

16

Week Eleven: Baggage Claim

3 Rounds, 45 on/15 off, AMRAP (reps): Complete each exercise as follows: As many reps as possible in 45 seconds, then 15 seconds to transition to the next exercise. Complete all 10 exercises and take 1 minute of rest between rounds. Complete 3 rounds.

Front Raises (palms face up)
  Suitcase Squats
  Woodchoppers
  DB Swing
  Alternating Front Lunge w/Torso Rotation
  Devil's Press
  Tricep Kickbacks
  C-seated Shoulder Press
  Rear Delt Flies
  Cross Body Hammer Curls

17

Week Twelve: Warrior

5 Rounds: 50/40/30/20/10: Complete the following circuit 5 times, each round with fewer reps than the previous. Rounds will include reps as follows: 50 each, 40 each, 30 each, 20 each, 10 each.

Thrusters
  Zottman Curls
  Sumo Deadlift High Pull
  DB Sit ups
  DB Squeeze Press (in bridge position)

Chapter 6: Adapting the Program for Your Needs

No two people are exactly alike when it comes to fitness. Age, experience, goals, and physical conditions all play a role in determining what works best for you. This chapter is designed to help you tailor the 12-week strength training program to your unique needs, whether you're just starting, an experienced lifter, or someone with special considerations.

Modifications for Beginners

Starting a strength training program can feel overwhelming, especially if you're new to working out. The key to success is building confidence while focusing on proper form and manageable progressions.

1. **Start Light and Focus on Form:**For beginners, mastering exercise mechanics is more important than lifting heavy. Using lighter weights or even bodyweight allows you to build a foundation without risking injury.

2. **Use Simplified Variations:**Certain exercises may feel intimidating or too challenging initially. For example:

- Perform knee push-ups instead of full push-ups.
- Avoid jumping during burpees

1. **Reduce Workout Volume:**Beginners don't need as much volume as more advanced lifters to see progress. Instead of completing 5 rounds of the workout, start with just two. You can also decrease the reps if necessary.
2. **Take Longer Rest Periods:**If you're new to strength training, your muscles may fatigue quickly. Allow yourself extra time to recover between sets—up to 90–120 seconds—so you can perform each exercise with proper form.
3. **Focus on Consistency:**Consistency is more important than intensity at this stage. Aim to complete all three weekly sessions, even if that means adjusting the intensity or duration. Showing up consistently builds the habit, which is essential for long-term success.

Special Considerations: Age, Gender, and Health Conditions

Strength training is for everyone, but individual circumstances can influence how you approach the program.

1. **Adapting for Age:**

- **Younger Lifters (Teens):** Focus on learning proper form and building a solid foundation. Avoid maximal lifts until you've developed a base of strength and experience.

- **Older Adults (50+):** Strength training is crucial for maintaining muscle mass, bone density, and mobility as you age. Use controlled movements, prioritize joint-friendly exercises, and allow adequate recovery time. Include more warm-up and mobility work to prepare your body for lifting.

1. **Gender-Specific Considerations:**

- **Women:** Strength training is equally effective for men and women, but societal myths may deter women from lifting heavier. Embrace progressive overload and focus on your personal goals, whether they include building muscle, increasing strength, or improving athleticism.
- **Men:** Men tend to have higher testosterone levels, which can enhance muscle growth. This often encourages heavier lifting, but it's equally important to prioritize form and balanced training to avoid overworking certain areas (e.g., chest over back).

1. **Health Conditions and Injuries:**

- **Pre-Existing Conditions:** If you have issues like arthritis, high blood pressure, or diabetes, consult with a healthcare provider before starting the program. Strength training can often improve these conditions when done safely and with proper guidance.
- **Injury Modifications:** For those recovering from injury, avoid exercises that aggravate the affected area. Replace them with safer alternatives or use resistance bands for a

gentler option. For example, swap out barbell deadlifts for dumbbell Romanian deadlifts if back pain is a concern.
- **Mobility Restrictions:** Limited range of motion doesn't mean you can't train. Adjust movements to accommodate your current abilities, gradually increasing mobility over time.

Putting It All Together

The beauty of strength training lies in its adaptability. This program is a framework that can be tailored to your starting point, experience level, and unique circumstances. Beginners can build confidence and form, intermediate and advanced lifters can push boundaries, and individuals with special considerations can modify as needed.

The most important part of any program is that it fits your life, goals, and abilities. Don't be afraid to make adjustments and experiment as you go. Strength training isn't a one-size-fits-all endeavor—it's a personal journey. By adapting the program to meet your needs, you're ensuring that this journey is both effective and sustainable.

19

Chapter 7: Overcoming Challenges

Embarking on a strength training journey is exciting, but challenges are inevitable. Life gets busy, progress may slow, and moments of doubt can creep in. The key to long-term success lies in staying motivated, navigating plateaus and setbacks, and leaning on a solid support system. This chapter provides practical strategies to help you push through obstacles and keep your commitment to the 12-week program.

Handling Plateaus and Setbacks

Plateaus and setbacks are natural parts of any fitness journey. How you respond to them determines whether you continue progressing or lose momentum.

Recognizing Plateaus: A plateau occurs when your progress slows or stalls. This can manifest as a lack of strength gains, no visible changes in your physique, or feeling stuck in your routine. Plateaus are a signal to reassess and adjust.

Breaking Through Plateaus:

- **Increase Intensity:** Add weight to your exercises, increase the number of reps, or increase the duration of the workout.
- **Change Your Routine:** Incorporate new exercises or modify the order of your workouts. This challenges your muscles in different ways and prevents adaptation.
- **Focus on Recovery:** Ensure you're getting enough rest, sleep, and nutrition to support your training. Overtraining can lead to plateaus.

Reframing Setbacks: Injuries, illnesses, or life events may temporarily derail your progress. Instead of viewing setbacks as failures, see them as opportunities to learn and reset. A short break doesn't erase your progress—it's part of the journey.

Practice Patience: Progress isn't linear. Some weeks you'll make significant gains; other weeks, it may feel like nothing is changing. Trust the process and focus on consistency rather than immediate results.

Building a Support System

You don't have to go through your strength training journey alone. A strong support system can provide motivation, accountability, and encouragement when challenges arise.

1. **Finding a Workout Partner:**Training with a partner can boost motivation and help you stay accountable. A good workout partner will challenge you to push harder, celebrate your successes, and help you maintain a consistent schedule.
2. **Joining a Community:**

- **In-Person Communities:** Gyms, fitness classes, and local clubs are excellent places to meet like-minded individuals. Surrounding yourself with others who share similar goals can keep you inspired.
- **Online Communities:** Social media groups, fitness forums, and workout apps often have communities where members share progress, tips, and encouragement.

1. **Seeking Guidance from Professionals:**Personal trainers and coaches can provide tailored advice, correct your form, and help you overcome plateaus. Investing in expert guidance is especially valuable if you're new to strength training or have specific goals.
2. **Sharing Your Goals:**Let friends and family know about your commitment to strength training. Even if they aren't directly involved, their support and understanding can help you stay focused.

Staying Mentally Strong

Staying motivated isn't just about physical preparation—it's also about mental resilience.

1. **Set Small, Achievable Goals:**Break your 12-week program into smaller segments, such as four-week phases. Achieving short-term goals provides frequent wins and keeps you motivated.
2. **Develop a Positive Mindset:**Replace negative thoughts with affirmations. Instead of saying, "I can't do this," tell yourself, "I'm getting stronger every day."
3. **Embrace the Journey:**Remember that fitness is a lifelong

endeavor. Enjoy the process of becoming stronger and healthier, and don't rush to achieve your ultimate goals.

Putting It All Together

Motivation ebbs and flows, but with the right strategies, you can navigate challenges and stay on course. Consistency, adaptability, and a strong support system are your greatest allies in this journey.

When life gets busy, remember that even small efforts add up. When plateaus hit, see them as opportunities to grow. And when setbacks arise, know that they're temporary.

Strength training is more than just physical exercise—it's a journey of resilience, growth, and self-discovery. By staying motivated and embracing challenges, you'll not only transform your body but also build the discipline and mental strength to tackle anything life throws your way.

20

Conclusion: Reflecting on Your Journey and Planning Your Next Steps

Congratulations! Completing a 12-week strength training program is no small feat. You've dedicated time, effort, and determination to transform your body and improve your overall health. As you reach the end of this chapter in your fitness journey, it's time to reflect on what you've accomplished, celebrate your success, and plan the next steps to maintain and build on the progress you've made.

Reflecting on Your Journey

Take a moment to think about where you started. Perhaps you were new to strength training, uncertain of what to expect. Maybe you had specific goals like building muscle, losing fat, or improving your overall fitness. Whatever your starting point, you've worked through challenges, stayed consistent, and come out stronger—physically and mentally.

What You've Achieved: Over the past 12 weeks, you've likely seen measurable improvements, such as:

- Increased strength and endurance.
- Improved muscle tone and definition.
- Enhanced energy levels and confidence.

These achievements are a testament to your hard work and the power of consistent effort.

Lessons Learned: Strength training isn't just about lifting weights; it's also about personal growth. Reflect on the lessons you've learned, such as:

- The importance of discipline and consistency.
- How to listen to your body and adapt to its needs.
- The value of patience and incremental progress.

Celebrating Wins: No matter how big or small, celebrate your accomplishments. Did you hit a personal best in a particular workout? Stick to your schedule despite a busy week? Overcome a setback? Recognize these moments as milestones in your journey.

Conclusion: The Start of Something Bigger

Completing this program is a significant accomplishment, and also a stepping stone to a lifetime of fitness and well-being. You've built strength, discipline, and resilience that will serve you far beyond the gym.

As you move forward, remember that your fitness journey is uniquely yours. Whether you continue to build on this program, explore new fitness challenges, or simply maintain the strength you've gained, the habits and knowledge you've developed will empower you to lead a healthier, more fulfilling life.

The possibilities are endless. Keep lifting, keep learning, and keep pushing toward your best self. This is just the beginning.

21

Exercise Glossary

Alternating Front Lunge with Torso Rotation

- **How to Do It:** Hold a dumbbell or medicine ball with both hands at chest height. Step forward into a lunge, then rotate your torso toward the side of your front leg. Rotate back to center as you return to standing. Alternate legs.
  - **Tip:** Keep your core engaged and movements controlled during the rotation.

Arnold Press

- **How to Do It:** Hold a dumbbell in each hand at shoulder height with palms facing you. As you press the weights overhead, rotate your wrists so your palms face forward at the top. Lower the weights and rotate your wrists back to the starting position.
- **Tip:** Perform the motion slowly and focus on smooth transitions between the rotation and press.

Bench Press (On Floor in Bridge Position)

- **How to Do It:** Lie on your back with feet flat and knees bent. Push through your heels to lift your hips into a bridge position. Hold dumbbells at chest level, press them straight up until arms are fully extended, then lower back down.
- **Tip:** Keep your core engaged to maintain stability in the bridge.

Bent Over Rows

- **How to Do It:** Hold a dumbbell in each hand, hinge forward at your hips, and let the weights hang toward the floor. Pull the dumbbells toward your torso by bending your elbows, then lower them back down.
- **Tip:** Keep your back straight and avoid rounding your shoulders.

Bicycle Crunches

- **How to Do It:** Lie on your back with your hands behind your head and legs lifted, knees bent. Alternate bringing your right elbow toward your left knee while extending your right leg, then switch sides.
- **Tip:** Keep your movements controlled and avoid pulling on your neck.

Box Jumps

- **How to Do It:** Stand facing a sturdy box or platform. Bend your knees slightly and swing your arms for momentum

as you jump onto the box. Land softly on the balls of your feet with your knees slightly bent. Step down carefully and repeat.
- **Tip:** Ensure the box is stable and appropriate for your fitness level.

Bulgarian Split Squats

- **How to Do It:** Stand a few feet in front of a bench and rest one foot on the bench behind you. Hold a dumbbell in each hand (optional) and lower into a lunge by bending your front knee. Push through your front heel to return to standing.
- **Tip:** Keep your torso upright and avoid letting your front knee go past your toes.

Burpees

- **How to Do It:** Start standing, drop into a squat, place your hands on the ground, and jump your feet back into a plank. Perform a push-up, jump your feet back toward your hands, and explosively jump up with your arms overhead.
- **Tip:** Move at a steady pace and modify by skipping the push-up or jump if needed.

C-Seated Lateral Raises

- **How to Do It:** Sit on the floor in a "C" shape with your torso slightly reclined and legs bent. Hold a dumbbell in each hand and lift your arms out to the sides until they reach shoulder height, then lower back down.

- **Tip:** Keep a slight bend in your elbows and engage your core to maintain balance.

C-Seated Shoulder Press

- **How to Do It:** Sit on the floor in a "C" shape with your torso slightly reclined and legs bent. Hold a dumbbell in each hand at shoulder height with palms facing forward. Press the dumbbells overhead until your arms are fully extended, then lower them back to shoulder height.
- **Tip:** Engage your core to maintain the reclined position and avoid arching your lower back.

Cleans

- **How to Do It:** Start with a dumbbell or barbell on the floor. Using your hips and legs, explosively lift the weight up to shoulder height in one smooth motion, keeping the barbell close to your body or guiding the dumbbell.
- **Tip:** Use your legs and hips to generate power, not just your arms.

Cross Body Curls

- **How to Do It:** Hold a dumbbell in each hand. Curl one dumbbell across your body toward the opposite shoulder, then lower it. Alternate sides.
- **Tip:** Keep your elbows close to your sides.

Curl & Press

- **How to Do It:** Hold a dumbbell in each hand. Perform a bicep curl, then press the weights overhead. Lower back down and repeat.
- **Tip:** Avoid arching your back during the overhead press.

Curtsy Lunges

- **How to Do It:** Stand tall and step one leg diagonally behind the other, lowering into a lunge. Return to the starting position and alternate legs.
- **Tip:** Keep your front knee aligned over your ankle for stability.

Devil's Press

- **How to Do It:** Start in a standing position holding a dumbbell in each hand. Drop into a burpee by placing the dumbbells on the ground, kicking your feet back into a plank, and performing a push-up. Jump your feet back toward your hands, then explosively lift the dumbbells overhead in a snatch-like motion. Return to standing and repeat.
- **Tip:** Move fluidly through the sequence, keeping your core tight during the plank and push-up.

Diamond Push-Ups

- **How to Do It:** Get into a push-up position with your hands forming a diamond shape under your chest. Lower your chest to your hands, then push back up.
- **Tip:** Keep your core tight and elbows close to your sides.

Dumbbell Curls

- **How to Do It:** Hold a dumbbell in each hand with arms by your sides. Alternate curling one dumbbell up while keeping the other stationary.
- **Tip:** Avoid using momentum—focus on your biceps.

Dumbbell Deadlifts

- **How to Do It:** Hold a dumbbell in each hand in front of your thighs. Hinge at your hips, lowering the dumbbells toward the floor while keeping your back straight. Stand back up by driving through your heels and extending your hips.
- **Tip:** Avoid rounding your back and focus on hip movement, not bending at the waist.

Dumbbell Snatch (DB Snatch)

- **How to Do It:** Place a dumbbell on the floor. With one hand, bend your knees and hinge your hips to grab the weight. In one explosive motion, pull the dumbbell up and overhead, keeping it close to your body. Lower it back down and switch sides.
- **Tip:** Focus on driving power through your hips and legs.

Dumbbell Step-Ups

- **How to Do It:** Hold a dumbbell in each hand and stand in front of a bench or platform. Step one foot onto the bench, driving through your heel to lift your body up. Bring the other foot up to stand fully on the platform. Step back down one foot at a time and alternate legs.

- **Tip:** Keep your torso upright and avoid leaning forward.

Dumbbell Squats

- **How to Do It:** Hold a dumbbell in each hand by your sides. Stand with feet shoulder-width apart and lower into a squat by bending your knees and hips. Push through your heels to return to standing.
- **Tip:** Keep your chest up and avoid letting your knees cave inward.

Dumbbell Swings (DB Swings)

- **How to Do It:** Hold one dumbbell with both hands and stand with feet shoulder-width apart. Hinge at your hips, swinging the dumbbell back between your legs. Thrust your hips forward to swing the dumbbell up to chest height. Control the descent and repeat.
- **Tip:** Focus on using your hips and glutes to generate momentum, not your arms.

Farmer's Carries

- **How to Do It:** Hold a heavy dumbbell or kettlebell in each hand by your sides. Stand tall with your shoulders back and core engaged, then walk a specified distance or for a set time.
- **Tip:** Keep your steps steady and avoid leaning to one side.

Flutter Kicks

- **How to Do It:** Lie on your back with your legs straight and hands under your hips for support. Lift your legs a few inches off the ground and alternate small, quick kicks.
- **Tip:** Keep your lower back pressed into the floor.

Front Raises (Palms Face Up)

- **How to Do It:** Hold a dumbbell in each hand with palms facing upward. Start with arms extended downward in front of your thighs. Lift the dumbbells straight up to shoulder height, keeping your arms extended, then lower back down.
- **Tip:** Avoid swinging or using momentum. Engage your shoulders and core for control.

Goblet Squats

- **How to Do It:** Hold a dumbbell or kettlebell at chest height with both hands. Stand with feet shoulder-width apart and lower into a squat, keeping the weight close to your chest. Push through your heels to return to standing.
- **Tip:** Keep your chest lifted and knees aligned over your toes.

Hammer Curls

- **How to Do It:** Hold a dumbbell in each hand with palms facing each other. Curl the weights up while keeping your wrists in a neutral position, then lower.

- **Tip:** Focus on controlled movements without swinging.

Hip Bridges

- **How to Do It:** Lie on your back with knees bent and feet flat on the floor. Push through your heels to lift your hips off the ground, forming a straight line from shoulders to knees. Lower back down and repeat.
- **Tip:** Squeeze your glutes at the top for maximum activation.

Jump Squats

- **How to Do It:** Perform a squat, then explode upward into a jump. Land softly and immediately go into the next squat.
- **Tip:** Use your arms for momentum and absorb the landing with bent knees.

Kettlebell Swings

- **How to Do It:** Stand with feet shoulder-width apart and hold a kettlebell with both hands. Hinge at your hips, swing the kettlebell back between your legs, then thrust your hips forward to swing the kettlebell up to shoulder height. Control the descent and repeat.
- **Tip:** Use your hips, not your arms, to generate momentum.

Knee-to-Chest Kickouts

- **How to Do It:** Sit on the floor with your hands behind you for support. Pull your knees to your chest, then extend your legs straight out without letting your feet touch the ground. Repeat.

- **Tip:** Maintain control and avoid leaning too far back.

Medicine Ball Slams

- **How to Do It:** Hold a medicine ball with both hands overhead. Explosively slam the ball into the ground, bending your knees slightly as you do so. Pick up the ball and repeat.
- **Tip:** Engage your core and use your entire body to generate power.

One-Leg Up Push-Ups

- **How to Do It:** Get into a push-up position with one leg lifted off the ground. Perform a push-up, keeping your core engaged and hips level. Alternate legs every 5–10 reps.
- **Tip:** Lower your chest fully and avoid sagging your hips.

Overhead Medicine Ball Squats

- **How to Do It:** Hold a medicine ball overhead with both hands. Perform a squat while keeping the ball lifted and your core engaged. Return to standing.
- **Tip:** Avoid letting the ball drift forward as you squat.

Plank to Push-Ups

- **How to Do It:** Start in a forearm plank position. Press one hand into the ground, followed by the other, to push up into a high plank. Lower back down to your forearms one arm at a time.

- **Tip:** Keep your body straight and avoid rocking your hips. Alternate the lead arm to work both sides evenly.

Pullovers

- **How to Do It:** Lie on a bench with a dumbbell held with both hands above your chest. Keeping your arms slightly bent, lower the weight back and over your head until you feel a stretch, then bring it back to the starting position.
- **Tip:** Keep your core engaged and avoid arching your lower back.

Pulsating Squats

- **How to Do It:** Lower into a squat position, then pulse up and down a few inches while staying in the squat. Perform small, controlled movements without fully standing up.
- **Tip:** Keep your weight in your heels and maintain a neutral spine.

Push Presses

- **How to Do It:** Hold a dumbbell in each hand at shoulder height. Slightly bend your knees and use your legs to drive the dumbbells overhead. Lower them back to shoulder height and repeat.
- **Tip:** Keep your core tight and avoid overarching your back.

Rear Delt Fly

- **How to Do It:** Hold a dumbbell in each hand and hinge forward at your hips, letting your arms hang toward the floor with palms facing each other. Keeping a slight bend in your elbows, lift the weights out to the sides until they are at shoulder height, then lower back down.
- **Tip:** Focus on squeezing your shoulder blades together at the top and keep your back straight.

Renegade Rows

- **How to Do It:** Get into a high plank position with a dumbbell in each hand. Row one dumbbell to your torso by bending your elbow, keeping your core tight to avoid twisting. Lower the dumbbell and repeat on the other side.
- **Tip:** Keep your hips steady and feet slightly wider for stability.

Shoulder Press

- **How to Do It:** Hold a dumbbell in each hand at shoulder height with palms facing forward. Press the weights overhead until your arms are fully extended, then lower back to shoulder height.
- **Tip:** Avoid shrugging your shoulders; keep them relaxed.

Skull Crushers

- **How to Do It:** Lie on a bench holding a dumbbell in each hand. Extend your arms above your chest, then bend your elbows to lower the weights toward your forehead. Extend back up.

- **Tip:** Move only your forearms; keep your upper arms stationary.

Suitcase Squats

- **How to Do It:** Hold a dumbbell in each hand by your sides, like carrying suitcases. Stand with feet shoulder-width apart. Lower into a squat by bending your knees and hips, then push through your heels to stand back up.
- **Tip:** Keep your chest up and weights close to your sides.

Sumo Deadlift High Pull

- **How to Do It:** Stand with feet wider than shoulder-width apart and toes pointed outward. Hold a dumbbell or barbell with both hands. Perform a sumo deadlift by hinging at your hips and lowering the weight toward the floor. As you stand back up, pull the weight up to chest height with elbows flaring outward. Lower the weight back down and repeat.
- **Tip:** Keep your back straight during the deadlift and drive power from your legs and hips into the upward pull.

Thrusters

- **How to Do It:** Hold a dumbbell in each hand at shoulder height with palms facing inward. Lower into a squat, then explosively stand up, pressing the dumbbells overhead in one fluid motion. Lower the dumbbells back to shoulder height as you descend into the next squat.
- **Tip:** Use the momentum from your legs to help drive the

weights overhead, and keep your core tight throughout.

Tricep Dips

- **How to Do It:** Sit on the edge of a bench, hands gripping the edge. Slide off the bench and lower your body by bending your elbows, then push back up.
- **Tip:** Keep your shoulders down and avoid locking your elbows at the top.

Tricep Extensions

- **How to Do It:** Hold one dumbbell with both hands above your head. Lower the dumbbell behind your head by bending your elbows, then extend your arms back up.
- **Tip:** Keep your elbows close to your head.

Tricep Kickbacks

- **How to Do It:** Hold a dumbbell in each hand and bend forward at your hips. Keep your upper arms close to your torso as you extend your arms straight back. Return to the start and repeat.
- **Tip:** Keep your core engaged and avoid swinging the weights.

Turkish Get-Ups

- **How to Do It:** Lie on your back holding a dumbbell or kettlebell in one hand above your chest. Bend the same-side knee, plant the foot, and use your free hand to prop

yourself up into a seated position. Push up into a lunge and stand while keeping the weight overhead. Reverse the steps to return to the start.
- **Tip:** Perform each step slowly and with control, focusing on balance.

V-Ups

- **How to Do It:** Lie on your back with arms extended overhead and legs straight. Simultaneously lift your arms and legs to form a "V" shape, reaching your hands toward your feet. Lower back down and repeat.
- **Tip:** Engage your core throughout the movement.

Walking Lunges

- **How to Do It:** Step forward with one leg, lowering your back knee toward the ground while keeping your front knee above your ankle. Push through your front foot to step forward into the next lunge with the other leg.
- **Tip:** Keep your torso upright and engage your core.

Woodchoppers

- **How to Do It:** Hold a dumbbell or medicine ball with both hands. Start with the weight above one shoulder, then rotate your torso as you bring the weight diagonally down across your body toward the opposite hip. Return to the starting position and repeat. Switch sides.
- **Tip:** Engage your core and move in a controlled manner.

Zottman Curls

- **How to Do It:** Hold a dumbbell in each hand with palms facing upward. Curl the dumbbells to your shoulders, then rotate your wrists so your palms face downward. Lower the weights back to the starting position. Rotate your wrists back to the original position and repeat.
- **Tip:** Move slowly and focus on controlling both the upward and downward phases of the movement.

22

References

Adams, A. (n.d.). *Progressive Overload explained: Grow muscle & strength today.* https://blog.nasm.org/progressive-overload-explained

Atakan, M. M., Li, Y., Koşar, Ş. N., Turnagöl, H. H., & Yan, X. (2021). Evidence-Based Effects of High-Intensity Interval Training on Exercise Capacity and Health: A Review with Historical Perspective. International Journal of Environmental Research and Public Health, 18(13), 7201. https://doi.org/10.3390/ijerph18137201

Evidence mounts on the benefits of strength training. (2024, March 5). News. https://www.hsph.harvard.edu/news/hsph-in-the-news/strength-training-time-benefits/

Hughes, D. C., Ellefsen, S., & Baar, K. (2017). Adaptations to endurance and strength training. *Cold Spring Harbor Perspectives in Medicine, 8*(6), a029769. https://doi.org/10.1

101/cshperspect.a029769

The difference between strength training and hypertrophy training. (2024, February 25). WebMD. https://www.we bmd.com/fitness-exercise/difference-between-strength-hypertrophy

Weight-training do's and don'ts. (n.d.). Mayo Clinic. https://www.mayoclinic.org/healthy-lifestyle/fitness/in-depth/weight-training/art-20045842